I0407810

Cinnamon Essential Oil

Benefits, Properties, Applications, Studies & Recipes

by Ann Sullivan

Published in USA by:

Ann Sullivan
217 N. Seacrest Blvd #9
Boynton Beach
FL 33425

© Copyright 2015

ISBN-13: 978-1545129593
ISBN-10: 1545129592

TABLE OF CONTENTS

Introduction

First things first, Essential Oils are natural and organic. They are derived from the significant compounds found in the plants that possess them. Seeds, bark, flower petals, stems and roots, as well as other functional parts of the plant, can all be used to extract Essential Oils from a given plant. All of us have experienced the aromatic properties of the plants that provide Essential Oils, even if we are completely unaware of what was taking place when it happened. Remember the last time you bought, or received, a dozen roses? That beautiful aroma exploding from the roses, is just a part of the aromatic properties and qualities of the Essential Oils that can be extracted from that particular flower. In conjunction with providing specific smells to certain plant species, Essential Oils also offer plants a layer of protection against diseases and possible predators. They also have a significant role to perform in the pollination procedures of the associated plant species.

Essential Oils are not water based. They are actually phytochemicals consisting of the powerful fragrant compounds of the plant. Phytochemicals are the compounds that occur naturally within the plant itself. This means that there are no synthetic additives, which are common in conventional medicines. Essential Oils are fat soluble; however they do not possess the same fatty acids or lipids associated with animal or vegetable oil products. Essential Oils are extremely clean, pure products that absorb into the skin almost immediately upon being touched. Essential Oils are translucent when unadulterated and have a color range that spans from crystal clear to a deep and vibrant blue hue.

Here is an experiment you can try at home. Take a fresh lemon and slice it in half. Peel the rind from the fruit and squeeze it between your hands. That aromatic fruity smelling residue left behind is chock full of ingredients used to make Essential Oils.

Essential Oils should not be confused with fragrance producing oils or perfumes. Essential Oils are natural and organic and are taken directly from the plant. Perfumes and fragrance oils are either artificially created, or manufactured with synthetic solutions and do not possess the same therapeutic properties as Essential Oils. Essential Oils are super concentrated substances, which means that a very little, usually a drop or two, will go a long way. The aromas and chemical compounds associated with Essential Oils allow them to provide therapeutic benefits for both physical and psychological procedures.

Essential Oils are offered by a number of manufacturers and distributors around the world. They vary in price and quality, which is determined by a number of different factors. The country of origin for the plant species being used, how rare the botanical is, how much oil can be produced by a specific plant, growing climate present for the plants, and standards applied by the distiller/manufacturer, will all play a very important role in determining price and effectiveness of the Essential Oils being produced.

Essential Oils are generally sold in small bottles or vials separately, or in slightly larger containers consisting of Essential Oil blends. The benefit of buying blends is that you can eliminate the need to purchase all Essential Oils separately. The disadvantage of buying blends is that you have no control of the mixture.

Chapter 3 will further detail past scientific research on cinnamon essential oil.

Now, let's get down to it – **Essential Oil 101: the Basics of Cinnamon.**

Summary: Cinnamon Bark, or Cinnamomum zeylanicum, is in the Cassia family, and so has similar properties. High quality cinnamon oil comes from Southeast Asia and, depending on which is processed – the tree's leaves or bark – the potential properties of cinnamon oil may vary.

Description: Cinnamon bark oil is commonly extracted through steam distillation. The bark is most often used. The oil is golden brown or yellow in color, oily in consistency, and has a strong spicy cinnamon scent.

Uses: Beyond those applications previously mentioned, additional uses for cinnamon bark essential oil include strengthening the body's natural defenses against of exhaustion, lice, rheumatism, constipation, flatulence, low blood pressure, and scabies. When it comes to mood and emotion, cinnamon bark can help relieve stress and exhaustion.

Properties: Antioxidant, antibiotic, antifungal, anti diarrhea, antibacterial, antiviral, antiseptic, astringent, hypoglycemic, emmenagogue, expectorant, digestive, stimulant and disinfectant.

Application: Dilute 1:3 with a carrier oil. You can apply topically, inhale directly, diffuse or use as a dietary supplement.

Safety Precautions: Cinnamon bark has been approved by the FDA for internal consumption and so can be used as a dietary supplement. Cinnamon bark should be heavily diluted if applied topically, as it may irritate the skin. If you are an alcoholic, are haemophiliac, or have prostate cancer or kidney or liver issues, do not use cinnamon bark.

Fun facts: Cinnamon bark is derived from the Greek word, "kinnamon."

Apart from Greece, cinnamon has its roots in many ancient civilizations, and the importation of cinnamon to Egypt is documented around 2000 BC. The product was so highly regarded that cinnamon was gifted to both monarchs and gods. An inscription on the temple of Apollo at Miletus mentions the gifts of cinnamon and cassia to the god of light, sun, truth and healing.

Chapter 1:
Benefits of Cinnamon Essential Oil

Cinnamon oil offers a number of therapeutic benefits; but you may be wondering what these benefits are. In this chapter, we'll take a closer look at the history of cinnamon and its many uses.

The Confusing Case of Cinnamon

Cinnamon is a spice of the genus Cinnamomum, which is acquired from the inner bark. Cassia is very closely related to cinnamon and is sometimes substituted for cinnamon in international commerce, although

Cinnamomum verum is commonly considered "true cinnamon." Dozens of other tree species produce spice products which are often substituted for this "true cinnamon" as well, and though they're not technically the same species, they are all related, being derived from the genus Cinnamomum and the family Lauraceae.

During the classical era, four varieties of cinnamon were differentiated and frequently confused with one another. The first was Cassia (Cinnamomum iners), which means "the peel of the plant," a quite literal name for the Arabian and Ethiopian bark which was scraped off the trees. The second was the "true cinnamon" (Cinnamomum verum), which originated in Sri Lanka. The third was Serichatum (Cinnamomum cassia), originating in China. And the last is Malabathrum (Cinnamomum tamala, and several other species), which literally means "dark-tree leaves," and originates in northern India.

The international importation of cinnamon to the Mediterranean was kept under wraps by the traders, in order that the suppliers might maintain a monopoly over the trade. In fact, Herodotus, the Greek historian now known as the "Father of History," believed that both cassia and cinnamon originated in Arabia and was protected by winged serpents. The spice was considered so sacred that even the magical immortal bird, the phoenix, chose to build its nest from cassia and cinnamon. To put these theories to rest, the origin story of true cinnamon is actually much less thrilling; it was simply a native crop cultivated in Sri Lanka, Burma, Bangladesh, and the Malabar Coast of India.

Alongside the Greeks, the Egyptians were also great advocates of cinnamon and cassia. They used it for aromatic purposes from the Hellenistic era forward. The spices were held in such high regards by the Egyptians that they were considered proper gifts to offer the rulers, as they were spices equal to royalty.

The Romans were also quite keen on this spice. In fact, cinnamon was such a hot commodity that Rome spent 100 million sesterces per year to transport it across the red sea, according to Pliny, the noted historian. A single Roman pound (327 grams) of cinnamon or cassia was then sold at upward of 300 denarii, which was equivalent to ten months' labor of the average worker. When his wife, Poppaea Sabina, passed away, the evil Emperor Nero burnt a year's supply of Rome's cinnamon for her funeral pyre in AD 65.

Cassia and cinnamon are also mentioned in the Hebrew Bible a number of times. The first mention is by Moses when he requested both for use in the holy anointing oil. Cinnamon also mentioned in Proverbs and the Song of Solomon; both refer to scenting with cinnamon as a perfume.

Cinnamon's true origin remained a mystery through the Middle Ages. The true source of cinnamon was first mentioned in Athar al-bilad wa-akhbar al-'ibad ("Monument of Places and History of God's Bondsmen") written by Zakariya al-Qazwini around 1270 AD.

The scale of production has since exploded. Globally,

cinnamon and cassia annually produce around 27,500-35,000 tons, of which cinnamomum verum (the "true" cinnamon) makes up roughly 7,500-10,000 tons. Sri Lanka produces the majority of this (about 80-90%), while Indonesia produces about two-thirds of the other species of Cinnamomum. China, Vietnam and India are also minor producers.

The cultivation of cinnamon is a long process. The tree grows for two years and is coppiced (cut from the stem), after which nearly a dozen fresh shoots are produced from these cut roots. The tree's stems must be processed directly following the harvest, as the inner bark needs to be wet. The outer bark is scraped off, and the branch is beaten with a hammer, which allows the inner bark to be scraped off in long rolls. The cinnamon strips that result are about a meter long, and they curl up naturally into the rolls you so often see. Once processed, the bark will dry within 4-6 hours, after which it is cut into 5-10 cm sticks and sold.

In Food

Flavoring foods, tea, and other beverages, cinnamon is highly versatile when it comes to its culinary uses. In Bangladesh and Pakistan, a favorite beverage combines cinnamon with cardamom, served hot. Cinnamon is also used as a spice for savory dishes, like lamb and chicken, in the Middle East and Turkey. Mexico is the main importer of cinnamon, and they use it, in particular, to prepare chocolate. The U.S. often combines cinnamon and sugar to flavor fruit products, breads, and cereals. Many dessert recipes see cinnamon as one of its constant ingredients, from candies to pies, doughnuts, and buns. It may come as a surprise that cinnamon can be used in pickling, as well.

If you're an alcohol connoisseur, then you probably know that cinnamon flavors a variety of alcoholic drinks. In Greece, a popular brandy offers "cinnamon liqueur," while in other European countries, Żubrówka remains a popular vodka flavoured with bison grass and cinnamon, while Maiwein is a white wine made of woodruff and flavored with – you guessed it – cinnamon.

Subspecies

Man has developed a number of different cinnamon strains and subspecies over the years, each of which offer unique properties and flavors, from spicy to sweet. We've identified some of the most popular subspecies below, all of which are frequently sold as cinnamon:

- Cinnamomum verum (originating in Sri Lanka; the "true cinnamon")

- Cinnamomum cassia (originating in China)

- Cinnamomum loureiroi (originating in Vietnam and Saigon; also known as Vietnamese cassia, Vietnamese cinnamon, or Saigon cinnamon)

- Cinnamomum burmannii (originating in Padang and Indonesia; also known as Padang cassia or Indonesian cinnamon)

Chemical Components

The essential oil of cinnamon is what creates the strong aromatic flavor; the oil composes 0.5 to 1% of cinnamon's composition. To produce the essential oil, the cinnamon bark is roughly beaten and macerated in sea water, after which the whole of it is distilled. Cinnamic aldehyde is what creates the pungent taste and scent, and, depending upon the species, it makes up around 90% of the bark's essential oil. Additional chemical components of cinnamon essential oil include ethyl cinnamate, linalool, eugenol (mostly in the leaves), beta-caryophyllene, and methyl chavicol.

It's important that these compounds remain intact, as they may help eliminate coughs, aid digestion, and fight against viruses, bacteria, fungi, and bodily parasites.

Main Properties of Cinnamon Essential Oil

Along with the antioxidant properties previously mentioned, cinnamon oil possesses antibacterial, antiviral, antifungal, anti-inflammatory, antiseptic, antidepressant, astringent, emmenagogue, hypoglycemic, expectorant and digestive properties. Cinnamon is well equipped to fight off any pathogen or wellness issue in the body's path.

Cinnamonum verum, as mentioned, is composed of

cinnamic aldehyde, ethyl cinnamate, linalool, eugenol (mostly in the leaves), beta-caryophyllene, and methyl chavicol. These components are what instill the enormously beneficial properties within cinnamon essential oil. We'll outline these properties below.

Antioxidant

Anything high in antioxidants – whether fruit, beans, or essential oils – is a powerful advocate for your body. Antioxidants both protect against free radicals and repair their damage. What are free radicals? Free radicals are destructive chemicals that invade your body, produced by substances both inside and out. Some free radicals (or oxidants) form through normal bodily reactions, like inflammation, metabolism and aerobic respiration. Other free radicals form outside the body, but enter it due to exposure. These include harmful pollutants, toxins, smoking, drinking alcohol, X-rays, and UV rays, just to name a few. Although our bodies produce their own antioxidants, these often become damaged as we grow older; thus, introducing antioxidants into our bodies allows these nutrients and enzymes to assist in chemical reactions which destroy the oxidants or free radicals. Cinnamon essential oil is a moderate antioxidant, aiming to detox the body of free radicals that lead to disease. The antioxidant properties of cinnamon were researched, and the results can be found here.

Antibacterial

Cinnamon's antibacterial properties make it a surefire aromatherapeutic oil; respiratory tract infections are staved off when airborne bacteria is eliminated from your common use environments. Read a study analyzing cinnamon's antibacterial properties here.

Antiseptic

When used as an antiseptic, cinnamon essential oil can inhibit the risk of infection in open wounds or other injuries.

Astringent

For those who do not know what an astringent is, it's a chemical compound that shrinks body tissues, which means it can aid skin issues and irritations, everything from acne to insect bites.

Antidepressant

When it comes to psychological issues, the uplifting scent of cinnamon combats negative thoughts and, thereby, depression.

Hypoglycemic

With its hypoglycemic properties, diabetics might turn to cinnamon to reduce and maintain their blood glucose levels.

Antiviral

The antiviral protection that cinnamon essential oil grants will essentially empower the immune system, building up a tougher wall of security that most colds, measles or mumps are unlikely to scale. This immune stimulant will ensure that your body is better prepared to protect against deadly viral infections.

Antifungal

While bacteria and viruses are plenty evil, fungi commonly lead to the most deadly infections, whether external or internal. Your ears, throat and nose are the most likely to become infected by fungi, the infections of which can be both excruciating and unsightly. If left untreated, fungal infections can kill, as they may spread to the brain. Cinnamon essential oil protects against these infections and more and is particularly effective against skin infections. A study examining cinnamon's antifungal properties can be found here.

Anti-inflammatory

External or internal inflammation can be reduced through the use of cinnamon essential oil. For instance, if you or your patient has swollen fingers from arthritis or a swollen knee from a sport's injury, oral application of cinnamon essential oil may decrease irritation or redness, while also soothing the pain that accompanies inflammation.

Emmenagogue

No need to look this one up. An emmenagogue is a menstrual stimulant for those with irregular menses. Cinnamon regulates hormones, which means that this emmenagogue can also delay and/or reduce the symptoms of menopause, which include hormonal and mood imbalance. A study about the emmenagogue properties of cinnamon can be read here.

Expectorant

Throat or respiratory infections can be staved off and relieved through the use of cinnamon essential oil. Acting as an expectorant, cinnamon breaks up and helps destroy the phlegm and mucus build ups that accompany sinuses or respiratory infections. Inflamed throat and lungs – and, thus, coughing – can also be relieved by the use of this oil.

Digestive

By boosting the production of absorptive enzymes, the digestibility of nutrients, and the secretion of digestive juices, cinnamon essential oil aids the digestive tract significantly, which can make a great impact on your overall wellness by increasing those nutrients you absorb from food.

Common Therapeutic Uses

Skin Infections

In combination with honey, cinnamon essential oil has long been used to support the body's defenses against acne and other skin conditions. The antimicrobial properties of the oil are especially effective when it comes to oily skin. For clearer skin, combine a teaspoon of honey with 2 drops cinnamon oil. Mix well and then apply to affected area (you may even consider using as a face mask). Allow to sit for 5-10 minutes, then rinse off. After several days of administration, you will see a marked difference.

Combating the Common Cold

For those of us who are susceptible to seasonal cold and flu viruses (so...everyone), providing your immune system with a reliable mechanism of defense can mean the difference between illness and wellness. According to a study published in the American Journal of Chinese Medicine, cinnamon essential oil does just that – it protects your immune system and provides strong support when you need it most. Cinnamon does this by combating bacterial and fungal growth, which is what often causes the common cold. A second study, published in the journal of Lab Medicine, discovered that cinnamaldehyde – a major component in cinnamon essential oil – has antiviral properties, making it an effective antidote against adenovirus.

Diabetes

A number of studies have been done on cinnamon's relationship to insulin and, thereby, diabetes. What these studies have found is that cinnamon helps boost insulin sensitivity, which aids diabetic management. Professor Paul David, from UC Davis, stated that cinnamon balances blood sugar levels with a 3-5% effectiveness – almost the same as diabetic pharmaceutical drugs. Moreover, reports were recently published by the Nutrition Research and Pharmacognosy Research which indicate that cinnamon supplemented in 1,500 mg dosages positively impacted not only insulin resistance, but liver enzymes, the lipid profile, and highly sensitive C-reactive protein in both diabetics and those non alcoholics with fatty liver disease (NAFLD), the latter of which is the primary cause of liver disease worldwide. One study on the part cinnamon plays in the body's defense against diabetes can be found here.

Allergies

Research in Egypt in 2006 analyzed cinnamon essential oil's capacity at repelling house mites, which have become some of the most invasive global allergens, according to the University of Kentucky College of Agriculture, Food and Environment, with allergies affecting around 45% of children. The research showed that amongst those oils tested, cinnamon was the deadliest at eliminating the house mites.

Candida Infections

The primary cause of urinary tract infection is Gram-negative E. Coli, which was amongst the 28 plant extracts studied by the Iran Journal of Medical Sciences. One of the most effective of the extracts was cinnamomum zeylanicum, which helped inhibit UTI's in those who supplemented it in their diet.

Aiding in Digestion

Digestive issues negatively impact many around the world. Cinnamon's antimicrobial properties help its patients to eliminate these issues. According to several studies, cinnamon essential oil is highly effective at support the body's defenses against E. coli infections, in particular. 2-3 cups of cinnamon tea a day can help relieve stomach issues, everything from cramps to indigestion. Combined with chamomile or ginger, the application will have an even stronger impact.

Promoting Energy

Due to its previously mentioned stabilizing ability when it comes to insulin and blood sugar, cinnamon has long been used to stimulate and sustain energy. In Chinese folk medicine, the oil was particularly used to stimulate "Qi," the most vital energy. Diffuse cinnamon essential oil in your room or have a cup of cinnamon tea. Combine either with peppermint, and you'll have a winning combination when it comes to energy boosting.

Safety Precautions & Common Applications

Safety

Some adverse effects may evolve when using pure essential oils. Some essential oils should not be used when pregnant, for example, as they may cause miscarriage. Allergic reactions, too, may occur, especially when applied topically. Always administer an allergy test before committing fully to topical application. When used with other medications, essential oils may react negatively. If you are on any current prescription medications or have a chronic illness, such as high blood pressure, epilepsy or liver disease, then researching the effects of essential oils against your own personal medical history will eliminate any potentially problematic issues.

Cinnamon bark has been approved by the FDA for internal consumption and so can be used as a dietary supplement. Cinnamon bark should be heavily diluted if applied topically, as it may irritate the skin. If you are an alcoholic, are haemophiliac, or have prostate cancer or kidney or liver issues, do not use cinnamon bark. Dilute 1:3 with a carrier oil. You can apply topically, inhale directly, diffuse or use as a dietary supplement.

Blends

Oftentimes, essential oils are manufactured as blends

of several pure oils. For instance, the protective blend is a mix of cinnamon, clove, rosemary, and eucalyptus. This blend can be used to boost the immune system to help support the body's defenses against colds, viruses and flus. The downside to blends is that the more oils added to the mix, the higher the probability the user may react negatively to the blend if he/she is prone to allergies. There is also the possibility of phototoxicity when working with blends.

Regardless of these possible effects, essential oils are a viable option for support the body's defenses against a number of conditions. Those looking to enhance the maintenance of their own personal wellness, or that of their families, should become educated on the uses of essential oils, their natural remedies and the methods of application. Only then can you begin building your kit of essential oils for everyday use and in a survival situation.

Chapter 2:
Recipes for Cinnamon Essential Oil

In this chapter, we'll offer various recipes for cinnamon essential oil, both for pure cinnamon supportive remedies and blends which incorporate the oil. For pure supportive remedies, we've provided the appropriate application and dosage to target specific ailments, from airborne bacteria to viral infections. When it comes to blends, herbalists and aromatherapists often combine cinnamon essential oil with frankincense, myrrh, ginger root, cardamom, coriander, black pepper, bergamot, orange, ylang ylang, clove bud, lavender, lemon, and Roman chamomile. We'll offer some fantastic supportive blending options in the second half of this chapter as well.

Pure Supportive Remedies

Airborne Bacteria

To stave off airborne bacteria during cold or flu season, diffuse cinnamon essential oil in a 1:3 ratio with your chosen carrier oil. You might also disinfect your car by applying a couple drops of cinnamon essential oil to a cotton ball and sticking it into the air conditioning vent, which will act as its own diffuser.

Aphrodisiac

Cinnamon has long been used to stimulate the libido. Diffuse regularly or dilute the cinnamon essential oil with a carrier oil and apply topically (to lower abdomen, not to genitals).

Bacterial Infections

Combat bacterial infections by diluting cinnamon essential oil with a carrier oil and applying topically over the affected area. You may also diffuse the oil for a similar effect.

Body Warmth

Cinnamon can serve to warm the body. Simply dilute cinnamon essential oil with a carrier oil and massage into chest, feet and around the neck.

Cooking

You can use cinnamon oil in cooking, as it's generally regarded as safe by the FDA. One drop to begin with; add more when necessary.

Diabetes

Regulate blood sugar and insulin levels by diluting cinnamon essential oil with a carrier oil and applying topically over the pancreas. You can also place 1-2 drops into a "00" capsule and ingest, or add a drop to each meal.

Diverticulitis

If you suffer from diverticulitis (inflammation of the colon), you can target the issue by diluting cinnamon essential oil with a carrier oil and massaging it over the abdomen every day.

Fatigue

Combat fatigue by diffusing cinnamon essential oil or adding a few drops to your bathwater. The warming oil will increase blood circulation, which will boost energy and brain function.

Fungal Infections

To strengthen the body's natural defenses against fungal infections, dilute cinnamon essential oil with a carrier oil and apply topically to affected area or rub into the soles of the feet. You can also diffuse the oil for a mild effect.

Immune Stimulant

Give your immune system a leg up by regularly diffusing cinnamon throughout your home, especially during cold and flu season. The scent also uplifts and boosts energy. Alternatively, you can add a couple drops to your bathwater or dilute with a carrier oil and apply topically. If you'd prefer the steam method, steam two drops of cinnamon essential oil in a pan of water, remove the steaming pan from the stove, pour into a bowl, place a towel over your head and inhale. If you don't feel it's done its job the first time, you can reheat that same water and use it once more without adding more oil.

Infection

To fight off infections, you can dilute cinnamon essential oil with a carrier oil and apply topically to the affected area or to the soles of the feat. You can also diffuse throughout the room, whichever application is more appropriate to your specific infection.

Insect Bites/Stings

Dilute cinnamon essential oil with a carrier oil and apply to the affected area to protect against infections and eliminate irritation.

Mold

Mold, mildew and fungus can cause a slew of wellness problems. Cinnamon will help rid of these fungi throughout your home. Apply a few drops directly, diffuse in the affected area, or place a few drops in your cleaning products.

Pancreas Support

Cinnamon oil helps regulate blood sugar and promotes pancreas function. To apply, dilute cinnamon essential oil with a carrier oil and apply topically over the pancreas or to the soles of the feet. You might also use it as a dietary supplement or add a drop to each meal.

Pneumonia

The antiviral properties of cinnamon essential oil will help combat illness, like pneumonia. To accelerate healing, diffuse cinnamon essential oil in the air.

Respiratory Issues

To fight respiratory issues, like asthma, dilute cinnamon essential oil with a carrier oil and massage over the chest and neck. You may also diffuse the oil for a similar effect.

Typhoid

To take down harsh bacterial infections, like typhoid,

dilute cinnamon essential oil with a carrier oil and apply topically as a full-body massage or to the soles of the feet. You may also diffuse the oil to clear up the bacteria.

Vaginal Infection

Apply cinnamon essential oil topically to strengthen the body's natural defenses against vaginal infection. Dilute the essential oil with a carrier oil and apply topically to the lower abdomen, massaging over the grown, but avoiding the genitals. Take care to use caution.

Viral Infection

Nearly any infection can be subdued with cinnamon essential oil. Dilute the essential oil with a carrier oil and apply topically over the affected area, to the soles of the feet, or use for a full-body massage.

Blends

Alert Mist Spray

Ingredients

- 20 drops Patchouli Essential Oil

- 35 drops Cinnamon Bark Essential Oil

- 35 drops Lime Essential Oil

- 110 drops Peppermint Essential Oil

- 4 ounces Distilled Water

Directions

Combine all ingredients in a dark colored glass spray bottle and, if drowsy when driving, spray in your car to stimulate alertness. Alternatively, you can use the blended oils in a car diffuser.

Chest Congestion

Ingredients

- 1 drop Cinnamon Essential Oil

- 1 drop Lemon Essential Oil

- 1 tsp Carrier Oil

Directions

To clear up chest congestion, combine all ingredients and massage into your chest three times a day.

Diabetic Support

Ingredients

- 8 drops Cinnamon Essential Oil

- 8 drops Clove Essential Oil

- 10 drops Thyme Essential Oil

- 15 drops Rosemary Essential Oil

- 2 ounces V-6

Directions

To help maintain insulin levels, combine all ingredients and apply topically to feet and over pancreas.

Energy Booster

Ingredients

- 10 drops Orange Essential Oil

- 10 drops Cinnamon Essential Oil

- 10 drops Black Pepper Essential Oil

Directions

Diffuse blend throughout your home to stimulate
energy.

Protective Blend

Ingredients

- 10 drops Rosemary Essential Oil

- 15 drops Eucalyptus Essential Oil

- 20 drops Cinnamon Bark Essential Oil

- 35 drops Lemon Essential Oil

- 40 drops Clove Bud Essential Oil

- 12 ounces Distilled Water

Directions

Combine all ingredients in a dark colored glass spray bottle and, during cold and flu season or if there's illness in the house, spray in all rooms to stimulate the immune system.

Fungal Infections

Ingredients

- 3 drops Grapefruit Essential Oil

- 2 drops Cinnamon Essential Oil

- 1 drop Basil Essential Oil

- 1 drop Patchouli Essential Oil

- ½ ounce Carrier Oil

Directions

To combat fungal infections, combine all ingredients and apply topically to affected area.

Gluten Intolerance Support

Ingredients

- 1 drop Cinnamon Bark Essential Oil

- 2 drops Grapefruit Essential Oil

- 2 drops Ginger Essential Oil

- 2 drops Lemon Essential Oil

Directions

To help strengthen the body's natural defenses against gluten intolerance, place all ingredients into a "00" capsule, and ingest 1 capsule a day.

Immune-Boosting Spray

Ingredients

- 4 ounces Distilled Water

- 60 drops Ginger Root Essential Oil

- 20 drops Cinnamon Bark Essential Oil

Directions

Combine all ingredients in a dark colored glass spray bottle and, during cold and flu season or if there's illness in the house, spray in all rooms to stimulate the immune system.

Immune-Boosting Topical Blend

Ingredients

- 5 drops Rosemary Essential Oil

- 8 drops Eucalyptus Essential Oil

- 10 drops Cinnamon Bark Essential Oil

- 18 drops Lemon Essential Oil

- 20 drops Clove Essential Oil

Directions

Combine all ingredients in a dark colored bottle and, during cold and flu season or if there's illness in the house, apply topically with a carrier oil to stimulate the immune system.

Poison Ivy

Ingredients

2 drops Cinnamon Bark Essential Oil

2 drops Thyme Essential Oil

13 drops Lemongrass Essential Oil

15 drops Rosemary Essential Oil

4 Tbsp Carrier Oil

Directions

To relieve poison ivy rash, combine all ingredients and apply topically to affected area.

Room Disinfectant

Ingredients

- 6 drops Cinnamon Bark Essential Oil

- 6 drops Pine Essential Oil(if available)

- 5 drops Juniper Berry Essential Oil

- 3 drops Clove Essential Oil

Directions

In a glass, marble, porcelain or ceramic aroma lamp, combine the essential oils with water. Diffuse the oils and deeply breathe in the vapors.

Stress-Reducing Massage Oil

Ingredients

- 1 Tbsp Carrier Oil

- 1 drop Lavender Essential Oil

- 3 drops Cinnamon Bark Essential Oil

- 3 drops Grapefruit Essential Oil

- 4 drops Fennel Essential Oil

- 4 drops Roman Chamomile Essential Oil

- 5 drops Melissa Essential Oil

Directions

In a small bowl or jar, combine oils, mixing until evenly distributed. Massage the oil into the shoulders, back and neck. Recommended for two-time use before a stressful event, 6 hours apart to help relieve anxiety.

Vapor Rub

Ingredients

- ½ cup Olive Oil

- 2 Tbsp Beeswax Pellets

- 20 drops Peppermint Essential Oil

- 20 drops Eucalyptus Essential Oil

- 10 drops Cinnamon Essential Oil

- 10 drops Rosemary Essential Oil

Directions

Combine ingredients in a mason jar and place jar in a saucepan with 1 inch of water. Over medium-low heat, mix beeswax and olive oil until melted and well blended. Remove from the stove and add in the essential oils, mixing until combined. Let cool completely before use. To apply, simply rub over chest, as you would a vapor rub.

Chapter 3:
Cinnamon Essential Oil Studies

Many studies have been done on essential oils to discover and prove their therapeutic qualities. In the case of the great number of cinnamon studies, many of the properties attributed to the essential oil (noted in this book and elsewhere) are quite often validated through the scientific research of accredited universities and published by accredited scientific journals. In this chapter, we'll discuss a small portion of these studies. It's important to note that research on essential oils is constant and evolving. Keep up with any recent research, as it may turn up even further valuable uses of these miracle oils.

Study 1 – Antimicrobial Properties

In this study published by the BMC Complementary and Alternative Medicine, the antimicrobial effects of cinnamon essential oil were examined, with the following results: "The main objective of this study was the phytochemical characterization of four indigenous essential oils obtained from spices and their antibacterial activities against the multidrug resistant clinical and soil isolates prevalent in Pakistan, and ATCC reference strains... Cinnamon (Cinnamomum verum)...was analyzed on GC/MS...Among all the tested essential oils, oil from the bark of C. verum showed best antibacterial activities against all selected bacterial strains in the MIC assay... Cinnamaldehyde was identified as the most active antimicrobial component present in the cinnamon essential oil which acted as a strong inhibitory agent in MIC assay against the tested bacteria. The results indicate that essential oils from Pakistani spices can be pursued against multidrug resistant bacteria."

In summary, this study showed that cinnamon bark oil was incredibly effective as an antibacterial agent against pathogenic strains Salmonella typhi (D1 Vi-positive), Salmonella typhi (G7 Vi-negative), Salmonella paratyphi A, Escherichia coli (SS1), Pseudomonas fluorescens and Staphylococcus aureus. Salmonella strains can cause an array of illnesses from typhoid fever to food poisoning. E. coli, as well, often results in serious food poisoning. Though a rare bacteria, P. Fluorescens may target those with compromised immune systems, such as cancer patients. And, lastly, S. aureus causes a whole host of illnesses and infections, including Staph infections, pimples, boils, impetigo, carbuncles, abscesses, scalded skin syndrome, and even pneumonia or meningitis. Cinnamaldehyde, one of the main chemical components in cinnamon essential oil, was found to be the most active prohibitory agent against these strains.

Reference
http://www.ncbi.nlm.nih.gov/pubmed/24119438]

http://www.ncbi.nlm.nih.gov/pmc/articles/PMC3853939/pdf/1472-6882-13-265.pdf]

Study 2 – Biocontrol in Fungal Contamination

In this study published by PLOS One, the antifungal effects of cinnamon essential oil were examined, with the following results: "Ochratoxin A (OTA) is a mycotoxin which is a common contaminant in grains during storage. Aspergillus ochraceus is the most common producer of OTA. Essential oils play a crucial role as a biocontrol in the reduction of fungal contamination. Essential oils namely natural cinnamaldehyde, cinnamon oil...were tested for their efficacy against A. ochraceus growth and OTA production by fumigation and contact assays. Natural cinnamaldehyde proved to be the most effective against A. ochraceus when compared to other oils...The study concludes that natural cinnamaldehyde, citral and eugenol could be potential biocontrol agents against OTA contamination in storage grains."

The research shows that cinnamon essential oil's antimicrobial activity – and particularly that of its active chemical component, cinnamaldehyde – showed biocontrol against Aspergillus ochraceus, which is a mold species that produces a highly invasive food-contaminating mycotoxin, ochratoxin A. A fungus commonly found in soil, agricultural goods, marine species and farmed animals, when consumed by humans, the fungus causes chronic immunosuppressive, neurotoxic, genotoxic, and carcinogenic issues. Furthermore, the fungi's airborne spores produce asthma in kids and other lung diseases. Consequently, the ability to control this fungi is imperative to human, animal, and agricultural health.

Reference
http://www.ncbi.nlm.nih.gov/pubmed/25255251]

http://www.ncbi.nlm.nih.gov/pmc/articles/PMC4178002/pdf/pone.0108285.pdf]

Study 3 – Antioxidant Properties

In this study published by ARYA Atheroscler 2013; Volume 9, Issue 5, the antioxidant effects of cinnamon essential oil were examined, with the following results: "Lipid oxidation is the main deterioration process that occurs in vegetable oils. This process was effectively prevented by natural antioxidants. Cinnamomum zeylanicum (Cinnamon) is rich with antioxidants. The present study was conducted to evaluate the effect of cinnamon on malondialdehyde (MDA) rate production in two high consumption oils in Iranian market...Compounds of cinnamon essential oil by GC-MS analysis such as cinnamaldehyde (96.8%), alpha-capaene (0.2%), alpha-murolene (0.11%), para-methoxycinnamaldehyde (0.6%) and delta-cadinen (0.4%) were found to be the major compounds...Essential oil of cinnamon considerably inhibited MDA production in studied oils and can be used with fresh and heated oils for reduction of lipid peroxidation and adverse free radicals effects on body."

Lipid peroxidation is when free radicals take electrons from cell membranes, which results in the oxidative degradation of lipids and significant cell damage. This causes a chain reaction, because whenever a normal cell is in contact with a radical, another radical is produced, which means the radicals begin to multiply at an exponential rate, the end result being carcinogenic or mutagenic. The natural antioxidant properties of cinnamon essential oil can inhibit the free radicals from damaging cell walls and multiplying.

Reference & Photo Credit:
http://www.ncbi.nlm.nih.gov/pubmed/24302936]

http://www.ncbi.nlm.nih.gov/pmc/articles/PMC3845693/
pdf/ARYA-09-280.pdf]

Study 4 – Menstruation

In this study published by Evidence-Based Complementary
and Alternative Medicine, the menstrual effects of
cinnamon essential oil were examined, with the following
results: "Dysmenorrhea is a common cause of sickness
absenteeism from both classes and work. This study
investigated the effect of aromatherapy massage on a group
of nursing students who are suffering of primary
dysmenorrhea... using the essential oils (cinnamon, clove,
rose, and lavender in a base of almond oil)...During both
treatment phases, the level and duration of menstrual pain
and the amount of menstrual bleeding were significantly
lower in the aromatherapy group than in the placebo group.
These results suggests that aromatherapy is effective in
alleviating menstrual pain, its duration and excessive
menstrual bleeding. Aromatherapy can be provided as a
nonpharmacological pain relief measure and as a part of
nursing care given to girls suffering of dysmenorrhea, or
excessive menstrual bleeding."

This study demonstrated the effectivity of cinnamon
essential oil against excessive menstrual bleeding and pain, a
condition known as dysmenorrhea. After massaging the
essential oil into the abdominal area during menses, both

the amount of bleeding and pain were significantly reduced.

Reference
http://www.ncbi.nlm.nih.gov/pubmed/23662151]

http://www.ncbi.nlm.nih.gov/pmc/articles/PMC3638625/
pdf/ECAM2013-742421.pdf]

Study 5 – Antibacterial Properties

In this study published by Iran J Med Sci, the antibacterial effects of cinnamon essential oil were examined, with the following results: "Brucella abortus is a gram-negative facultative intracellular bacterium that can cause a highly contagious disease in sheep, goats, cattle and one-humped camels. It is responsible for one of the most important zoonosis in human. The aim of this study was to evaluate the role of...Cinnamomum verum essential volatile oil extracts on human macrophages infected by B. abortus 544...Cinnamomum verum volatile oil at a concentration of 1% had the highest antibacterial activity against B. abortus 544 inside human macrophages...The results indicate that, among the five selected oil extracts, C. verum volatile oil applied either separately or in combination with other oil extracts had the most effective antimicrobial activity against Brucella."

As stated in the summary, although Brucella abortus primarily affects farm animals, it can be transmitted to humans. When it is, the bacteria produces a disease called brucellosis, also known as "Malta Fever," due to its initial discovery being in those soldiers living in Malta. Once infected by the pathogen, the disease can pass from acute to chronic, after which the host must deal with the consequences of the disease for life. These consequences include fatigue, joint pain, and headaches, while the acute symptoms include weight loss, fever, backache, headache, chills, and weakness. The effectivity of cinnamon essential oil against the human macrophages was high against Brucella, meaning it could potentially be used as a source of support against this chronic disease.

Reference
http://www.ncbi.nlm.nih.gov/pubmed/23115441]

http://www.ncbi.nlm.nih.gov/pmc/articles/PMC3470071/pdf/IJMS-37-119.pdf]

Study 6 – Diabetes

In this study published by Cardiovascular Diabetology, the antidiabetic effects of cinnamon essential oil were examined, with the following results: "This study was made to investigate the antidiabetic, antioxidant and hypolipidemic potential of Cinnamomum tamala, (Buch.-Ham.) Nees & Eberm (Tejpat) oil (CTO) in streptozotocin (STZ) induced diabetes in rats along with evaluation of chemical constituents...CTO (100 mg/kg and 200 mg/kg), cinnamaldehyde (20 mg/kg) and glibenclamide (0.6 mg/kg) in respective groups of diabetic animals administered for 28 days reduced the blood glucose level in streptozotocin induced diabetic rats...The results of CTO and cinnamaldehyde were found comparable with standard drug glibenclamide. In vitro antioxidant studies on CTO using various models showed significant antioxidant activity. In vivo antioxidant studies on STZ induced diabetic rats revealed decreased malondialdehyde (MDA) and increased reduced glutathione (GSH)."

This study shows the potential for cinnamon essential oil in strengthening the body's natural defenses against diabetes. The results demonstrated that cinnamon essential oil reduced blood glucose levels, along the same line as the standard diabetic drug glibenclamide.

Reference
http://www.ncbi.nlm.nih.gov/pubmed/22882757]

http://www.ncbi.nlm.nih.gov/pmc/articles/PMC3461457/pdf/1475-2840-11-95.pdf]

Study 7 – Colon Cancer

In this study published by the National Institutes of Health, the antioxidant effects of cinnamon essential oil on colon cancer cells were examined, with the following results: "Colorectal cancer (CRC) is a major cause of tumor-related morbidity and mortality worldwide. Recent research suggests that pharmacological intervention using dietary factors that activate the redox sensitive Nrf2/Keap1-ARE signaling pathway may represent a promising strategy for chemoprevention of human cancer including CRC. In our search for dietary Nrf2 activators with potential chemopreventive activity targeting CRC, we have focused our studies on trans-cinnamic aldehyde (cinnamaldeyde, CA), the key flavor compound in cinnamon essential oil. Here we demonstrate that CA and an ethanolic extract (CE) prepared from Cinnamomum cassia bark, standardized for CA content by GC-MS analysis, display equipotent activity as inducers of Nrf2 transcriptional activity...Taken together our data demonstrate that the cinnamon-derived food factor CA is a potent activator of the Nrf2-orchestrated antioxidant response in cultured human epithelial colon cells. CA may therefore represent an underappreciated chemopreventive dietary factor targeting colorectal carcinogenesis."

The study examined the use of cinnamon essential oil's chemical compound, cinnamaldehyde, as a strategy for chemoprevention in cancer, particularly in colorectal cancer. The study found that cinnamaldehyde activated the antioxidant response in cultured human epithelial colon cells, which means it can indeed serve as a chemopreventive dietary factor when fighting rectal cancer.

Reference:

http://www.ncbi.nlm.nih.gov/pubmed/20657484]

http://www.ncbi.nlm.nih.gov/pmc/articles/PMC3101712/pdf/nihms293405.pdf]

Chapter 4:
The Ins & Outs of Essential Oils

Where do essential oils come from?

Plants and plant species naturally produce essential oils for various reasons, one being to draw pollinator insects to them, another being to repel invading organisms (bacteria, animals). A number of chemical compounds compose each plant's essential oil, and the combination of these compounds is specific to each oil, which then instills in the oil its own unique properties. Essential oils can be harnessed from all sorts of plant components, including flowers, leaves, bark, fruit, roots, and resin. For instance, cinnamon oil is harnessed from bark, lemon oil from the peel, and lavender oil from lavender flowers. Certain plants can produce a few chemical variants of the same essential oil, which are acquired from different parts of the plant.

Some of these parts produce a large amount of oil, while others produce just a smidgen. The oil's quality and potency depends upon a number of factors, including the subspecies of the plant, its soil conditions, the time of year and even the time of day you harvest it.

How are essential oils extracted?

Essential oils can be extracted from plants through various methods, including pressing, distillation, solvent and maceration. Let's take a brief look at each:

Pressing Method

Commonly used with citrus fruit, the pressing method extracts the oil through a technique which involves pushing the fruit peels through a press. Oily fruits and plants are best suited for this technique. Orange oil, for example, is extracted from orange skins through the pressing method.

Distillation Method

This technique harkens back to the days of old-timey moonshiners, as the same sort of method used to create strong liquor can be used to extract essential oils. Using a still, boiled water and plant materials will create steam which is then cooled by coils and condensed into a combination of water and oil. This combination doesn't mix, so the oil can then be extracted from it.

Solvent Method

Through a multi-step process, certain plant and flower oils can be extracted using alcohol and other solvents, which extort the essential oil from the plant materials.

Maceration Method

When a "carrier" or fixed oil or lard is mixed with the plant material and set out in the sun, over a period of time, the carrier oil is infused with the plant's essence. Heat sources, other than the sun, are often used to speed the process. Throughout the process, more plant material is added to produce a more potent oil.

How do you use essential oils?

Although some studies about the effectiveness of essential oils are conducted by small companies or even individuals, a number of them are conducted by the food and cosmetic industries. In general, the pharmaceutical industry shows next to no interest in herbal medicine, primarily because there are few options to patent such products. Being as such, the product's lack of profitability results in a lack of research funding. Regardless, the historical uses of essential oils tell us what we need to know: these oils have been effectively administered for centuries. The therapeutic qualifications of essential oils can be plotted in the survival of the human race across cultures and generations.

Another reason that studies on essential oils have not resulted in much conclusive evidence as to their overall effectiveness is because definitive results are sometimes difficult to prove, as the quality of each batch of oil can vary for a number of reasons. One is that essential oils are impossible to standardize. As mentioned above, even the slightest variance in soil conditions and the time of harvesting – as well as innumerable other factors – will produce a different product quality and potency. In addition, essential oils are often obtained from various species of the same plant; Eucalyptus radiata and Eucalyptus globulus can both be used in the making of therapeutic-grade eucalyptus oil and, as a result, they may have slightly different properties and degrees of strength or effectiveness.

Just as there are a number of methods by which to extract essential oils, there are a number of methods to administer them therapeutically. The variety of chemical compounds in each essential oil means that their benefits and applications also vary across the board. Below are a few of these methods.

Topical Administration

Direct application of many essential oils works like a sponge, as skin sops up chemicals and other things (like sunlight, for instance). Topical application is best when you want to clear up an ailment on the skin's surface or in the underlying muscle tissue. When applying topically, you may either massage the oil into the skin or simply dab on the skin for therapeutic results. You might combine the essential oil with a carrier oil for topical use in order to dilute its potency. This is safer, as the oil is so concentrated. You may support your body's defenses against rash or muscle pain in this manner, but you should always test your patient for allergies before applying. Adverse effects are produced by natural chemicals as much as synthetic ones; poison ivy, for example.

To test for allergens, place a drop or two on your patient's inner forearm. If a rash develops within 12 to 24 hours, then the patient is allergic. In addition, phototoxicity – sun exposure resulting in an exacerbated burn – may be an issue when citrus oils are applied topically. So one must proceed with caution when applying essential oils using this method.

Inhalation Therapy

Commonly known as "aromatherapy", this essential oil application is effective for inner ailments, like sore throat or cold. In a steaming bowl of distilled or sterilized water, add a few drops of essential oil and, with a towel over your head, bend over the bowl and inhale. The towel captures the vapors, making the technique even more effective. Essential oils can also be placed in a diffuser or potpourri throughout a room to produce somewhat diluted therapeutic effects.

Ingestion

When using this method, proceed with caution. Direct ingestion of essential oils must be monitored and applied in small doses that are diluted in a tablespoon or more of any carrier oil – olive oil, for example. If you are unsure of dosage amounts, make a tea with the relevant herb instead. Although the effects of this diluted use may be weaker, this application is a better alternative than an overdose of essential oils.

What are the general benefits of using essential oils?

Replacement for Prescription Drugs

One practical benefit for using essential oils is, of course, their substitutive nature; they can replace Rx drugs, which is the ultimate reason to educate yourself on their administration and to begin stockpiling your essential oil supply. One of the potential threats of economic or social collapse is the lack of resources, and primarily the inability to procure prescription drugs. Being as such, finding suitable supplements should be a priority when preparing for the worst.

Their portability is also a major bonus when it comes to survival prepping. The fact that these ultra-concentrated oils take up little-to-no space makes toting them to your shelter all the simpler should the need arise. And, because essential oils are highly concentrated, the application used in most methods of administration requires only a drop or two of oil, which means that tiny bottle will be long-lasting.

Cost Effective Supplement

Though money may be the last thing on your mind when it comes to prepping for a survival situation (money may even be obsolete in the event of social collapse), it is worth noting that the expense of essential oils pales in comparison to prescription drugs. Essential oils are a cost effective supplement to prescription medicine.

No Expiration Date

Another benefit of essential oils is that they do not expire, neither do they have "proper storage" requirements. A number of medicines and medicinal products must be replaced every couple years, so this sets essential oils ahead of the pack when it comes to shelf life.

Versatility

Essential oils also offer great versatility. Apart from providing therapeutic benefits, essential oils can be repurposed for household and hygienic applications. For instance, if you're looking for something that might serve your dental hygiene needs in a time of crisis, the protective oil blend is your go-to essential oil. If you want to maintain your skin's tone and condition, frankincense and lavender will do the trick; the latter also serves as sunscreen, so you can inhibit sun damage as well.

When it comes to the house or shelter, you can use essential oils to deodorize, which will come in handy in a disaster scenario where things might start to smell fishy due to lack of proper utilities and care. For example, after the 2011 tsunami and the subsequent nuclear reactor meltdown in Japan, a nurse named Risa Nakahira used essential oils to deodorize and sanitize putrid public bathrooms in overpopulated evacuation facilities. As relief workers searched for survivors, often wading through debris and decay, Nakahira also deodorized their boots and masks using essential oils. The possibilities of these natural oils are endless.

They are also versatile when it comes to the range of patients they're capable of supporting. The wellness of everyone from your great grandfather to your infant baby can be fortified with the aid of essential oils in the appropriate dosage. They even come in handy when supporting the wellness of livestock or pets. From teething infants to dementia in the elderly, from teenagers with acne to dogs with urinary tract infections, essential oils can serve any patient with nearly any ailment.

Conclusion

Now that you know all about what cinnamon essential oil can do for you – where it originates, how it's extracted, its benefits and properties, and the different methods of administration – you can use it confidently to support the body's defenses against wellness issues and start to assemble a kit of essential oils for survival. Essential oils can be purchased online or at your local holistic treatment store. We always recommend using 100% Pure therapeutic grade oils.

The various benefits of essential oils and their properties are countless. To build your own kit, first focus on acquiring the essential oils which may bear more relevance to your wellness issues or the potential threats within your environment. In the event of a viral outbreak, for instance, cinnamon essential oil will be one of your more crucial oils due to their antiviral and immuno-supportive properties.

Used as a supplement or as your go-to for digestive issues, viral infections or immune-boosting agents, the application of cinnamon essential oil in medicine has survived for centuries and will survive centuries more. When it comes down to it, you don't need to rely on pharmaceuticals; essential oils, herbs, and plenty of other natural ingredients can be used to help support the body's natural defenses against any number of wellness issues, whether ailment or injury.

Essential oils are essential to your survival in the case of viral outbreak, social collapse or natural disaster because, when the SHTF, your access to pharmaceuticals will likely either be limited or eliminated altogether. Supplements to our modern-day standard will equate survival when no other option exists. And when it comes to a life-or-death situation, you can't let your wellness decline, no matter the state of the world.

Statements and research referenced in this educational work have not been evaluated by the Food and Drug Administration. Recommendations described are not intended to diagnose, treat, cure, or prevent disease. Products referenced in this presentation are safe to use and specifically formulated to support wellness.

DISCLAIMER AND/OR LEGAL NOTICES: Every effort has been made to accurately represent this book and it's potential. Results vary with every individual, and your results may or may not be different from those depicted. No promises, guarantees or warranties, whether stated or implied, have been made that you will produce any specific result from this book. Your efforts are individual and unique, and may vary from those shown. Your success depends on your efforts, background and motivation.

The material in this publication is provided for educational and informational purposes only and is not intended as medical advice. The information contained in this book should not be used to diagnose or treat any illness, metabolic disorder, disease or health problem. Always consult your physician or healthcare provider before beginning any nutrition or exercise program. Use of the programs, advice, and information contained in this book is at the sole choice and risk of the reader.